SOMATIC YOGA FOR WEIGHT LOSS

Stress Reduction And Weight Loss And The Powerful Connection Between Relaxation And Shedding Pounds With Somatic Yoga

CONTENT

INTRODUCTION

A. Understanding Somatic Yoga:

I. Definition and Principles of Somatic Yoga:

Somatic yoga is a holistic approach to yoga that emphasizes the internal experience of the body. Unlike traditional yoga, which often focuses on achieving specific postures or external alignment, somatic yoga encourages practitioners to tune into their own bodily sensations and movements. The word "somatic" derives from the Greek word "soma," meaning "living body," highlighting the practice's focus on the body's internal awareness and intelligence.

The principles of somatic yoga include mindful movement, sensory awareness, and self-regulation. Practitioners are guided to move slowly and consciously, paying close attention to how their bodies feel during each movement. This heightened awareness helps to release tension, improve flexibility, and foster a deeper connection between the mind and body.

II. How Somatic Yoga Differs from Traditional Yoga:

While both somatic yoga and traditional yoga aim to promote physical and mental well-being, their approaches are distinct. Traditional yoga often emphasizes the attainment of specific poses and sequences, with a focus on external form and alignment. In contrast, somatic yoga prioritizes the individual's internal experience, encouraging movements that feel natural and comfortable for the practitioner.

In somatic yoga, there is less emphasis on achieving a perfect posture and more on exploring movements that release muscular tension and enhance body awareness. This approach can be particularly beneficial for those who may find traditional yoga poses challenging or intimidating. By focusing on the body's internal sensations, somatic yoga creates a more personalized and accessible practice.

III. The Mind-Body Connection in Somatic Practices:

Central to somatic yoga is the concept of the mind-body connection. This connection refers to the interrelationship between our mental and physical states, where our thoughts, emotions, and bodily sensations influence one another. Somatic practices recognize that physical tension and pain are often linked to mental and emotional stress, and by addressing the body, we can also impact our mental and emotional well-being.

Somatic yoga techniques aim to heighten this mind-body awareness. Through mindful movement and sensory exploration, practitioners learn to listen to their bodies and respond to their needs. This can lead to greater self-awareness, emotional balance, and stress reduction. By fostering a deep sense of connection between the mind and body, somatic yoga helps individuals achieve a state of holistic wellness, which is essential for sustainable weight loss and overall health.

In the following chapters, we will explore how somatic yoga can be specifically tailored to support weight loss, incorporating mindful practices that promote physical, mental, and emotional well-being. By understanding and embracing the principles of somatic yoga, you will be equipped with the tools to embark on a transformative journey towards a healthier, more balanced life.

THE SCIENCE BEHIND SOMATIC YOGA AND WEIGHT LOSS

A. How Somatic Yoga Affects the Body:

I. Neuromuscular Re-education"

Somatic yoga focuses on reprogramming the brain's control over muscles through mindful movement, which is known as neuromuscular re-education. This process helps to:

1. Release Chronic Muscle Tension: By engaging in slow, controlled movements, somatic yoga helps to identify and release chronic muscle tension. This can improve flexibility and mobility, allowing for more efficient and

effective movement during physical activities.

2. Improve Posture and Alignment: Poor posture can lead to inefficient movement patterns and unnecessary strain on the body. Somatic yoga promotes better posture by teaching the body how to move more efficiently and align correctly, which can enhance overall physical performance and reduce the risk of injury.

3. Enhance Muscle Function: Through repeated practice, somatic yoga helps to fine-tune the communication between the brain and muscles. This results in improved muscle coordination and strength, which can support more

vigorous exercise routines and facilitate weight loss.

II. Stress Reduction and Its Impact on Weight:

Stress is a significant factor that can contribute to weight gain. Somatic yoga addresses this issue by:

1. Activating the Relaxation Response: Somatic yoga includes practices that activate the parasympathetic nervous system, which promotes relaxation and reduces the production of stress hormones like cortisol. Lower cortisol levels are associated with reduced abdominal fat and overall weight loss.

2.	Promoting Mind-Body Connection: By focusing on the present moment and bodily sensations, somatic yoga helps practitioners become more aware of their stress levels and how they manifest in the body. This heightened awareness can lead to better stress management strategies and healthier lifestyle choices.

3. Enhancing Sleep Quality: Stress often disrupts sleep, and poor sleep is linked to weight gain. The relaxation techniques in somatic yoga can improve sleep quality, thereby supporting weight loss efforts by allowing the body to recover and function optimally.

III. Improved Body Awareness and Mindful Eating:

One of the core principles of somatic yoga is cultivating a deep sense of body awareness, which can significantly influence eating habits:

1. Mindful Eating: By increasing awareness of hunger and satiety signals, somatic yoga encourages mindful eating. Practitioners learn to recognize when they are truly hungry and when they are full, which helps prevent overeating and promotes healthier food choices.

2. Emotional Eating Awareness: Many people eat in response to emotions rather than physical hunger. Somatic yoga helps individuals become more attuned to their emotional states and

develop healthier coping mechanisms, reducing the likelihood of emotional eating.

3. Better Food Choices: With improved body awareness, individuals are more likely to choose foods that nourish their bodies rather than those that provide only temporary comfort. This can lead to a more balanced diet and support long-term weight loss goals.

B. Scientific Evidence:

I. Studies Supporting Somatic Yoga for Weight Loss:

1. Research on Neuromuscular Re-education: Studies have shown that practices focusing on neuromuscular re-education can

improve muscle function and physical performance. For example, a study published in the Journal of Bodywork and Movement Therapies* found that somatic exercises improved flexibility and reduced pain in participants, suggesting potential benefits for weight loss efforts through enhanced physical activity.

2. Stress Reduction and Weight Loss: Research has consistently demonstrated the link between stress reduction and weight loss. A study in the Journal of Obesity highlighted that stress management techniques, including yoga, led to significant reductions in body weight and abdominal fat among participants.

3. indful Eating and Weight Loss: Numerous studies support the role of mindful eating in weight management. A review in the *Journal of the Academy of Nutrition and Dietetics* concluded that mindful eating interventions are effective in promoting weight loss and improving eating behaviors.

II. Testimonials and Case Studies:

1. Case Study: Sarah's Journey: Sarah, a 35-year-old mother of two, struggled with stress-induced weight gain for years. After incorporating somatic yoga into her routine, she reported not only a significant reduction in stress levels but also a steady weight loss of 15 pounds over six months. Sarah credits her success to the

increased body awareness and improved stress management she gained through somatic yoga.

2.   Testimonial: Mark's Transformation: Mark, a 45-year-old professional, faced chronic back pain and weight issues. Through regular somatic yoga practice, he experienced relief from his back pain and lost 20 pounds over a year. Mark attributes his weight loss to the neuromuscular re-education and mindful eating habits he developed during his somatic yoga sessions.

3. Case Study: Lisa's Mindful Eating: Lisa, a 28-year-old teacher, struggled with emotional eating. Somatic yoga helped her become more aware of her

emotional triggers and develop healthier coping strategies. Over eight months, Lisa lost 18 pounds and reported a more balanced relationship with food, thanks to the mindful eating practices she learned from somatic yoga.

By understanding the science behind somatic yoga and its impact on the body, it's clear how this practice can be a powerful tool for weight loss. The combination of neuromuscular re-education, stress reduction, and improved body awareness creates a holistic approach that not only supports weight loss but also promotes overall well-being.

GETTING STARTED WITH SOMATIC YOGA

Embarking on a journey with somatic yoga for weight loss is a transformative experience. This chapter will guide you through the initial steps to prepare your mind and body, introduce you to basic techniques, and help you establish a foundation for your practice. Let's begin by setting the stage for your success.

A. Preparing Your Mind and Body:

I. Setting Intentions for Weight Loss:

Before diving into the physical practice, it's essential to set clear and meaningful intentions.

Intentions are more than just goals; they are the guiding principles that shape your journey.

1. Reflect on Your Motivation: Take some time to ponder why you want to lose weight. Is it for improved health, increased energy, better mobility, or enhanced self-esteem? Understanding your 'why' can provide a strong motivational foundation.

2. Visualize Your Success: Close your eyes and imagine yourself having achieved your weight loss goals. How do you feel? What activities can you enjoy? Visualization can be a powerful tool to keep you motivated and focused.

3. Create Affirmations: Develop positive affirmations that resonate with your goals. Phrases like "I am becoming healthier every day" or "I honor my body with mindful movement" can reinforce your commitment.

4. Set Realistic Milestones: Break down your weight loss journey into achievable milestones. Celebrate each success, no matter how small, to maintain momentum and stay encouraged.

II. Creating a Conducive Environment for Practice:

Your environment plays a crucial role in supporting your somatic yoga practice. Here are some tips to create a space that fosters relaxation and focus:

1. Choose a Quiet Space: Select a location where you can practice without interruptions. This could be a dedicated room, a corner of your living space, or even an outdoor area.

2. Ensure Comfort: Use a yoga mat, blankets, or cushions to make your practice comfortable. Wear loose, breathable clothing that allows for freedom of movement.

3. Minimize Distractions: Turn off electronic devices or place them on silent mode. If possible, inform family members or housemates about your practice time to minimize interruptions.

4. Incorporate Elements of Nature: If feasible, practice near a window with natural light or

incorporate plants and natural materials into your space to enhance tranquility.

5. Create a Ritual: Establish a pre-practice routine that signals to your body and mind that it's time for yoga. This could include lighting a candle, playing soothing music, or performing a few minutes of meditation.

B. Basic Somatic Yoga Techniques:

Now that your mind and environment are prepared, let's explore some fundamental somatic yoga techniques to get you started.

I. Breathing Exercises:
Breath is the bridge between the body and mind. By mastering

breathing techniques, you can enhance relaxation, focus, and overall well-being.

1. Diaphragmatic Breathing: Sit or lie down comfortably. Place one hand on your chest and the other on your abdomen. Inhale deeply through your nose, allowing your abdomen to rise while keeping your chest still. Exhale slowly through your mouth. Repeat for several minutes, focusing on the rise and fall of your abdomen.

2. 4-7-8 Breathing: Inhale quietly through your nose for a count of 4. Hold your breath for a count of 7. Exhale completely through your mouth for a count of 8. This technique can help calm the nervous system and reduce stress.

3. Alternate Nostril Breathing: Sit comfortably and use your right thumb to close your right nostril. Inhale deeply through your left nostril. Close your left nostril with your right ring finger, release your right nostril, and exhale through it. Inhale through the right nostril, then switch and exhale through the left. Continue this pattern for several minutes.

II. Gentle Movements and Stretches:

Somatic yoga emphasizes gentle, mindful movements that increase body awareness and release tension.

1. Cat-Cow Stretch: Start on your hands and knees in a tabletop position. Inhale as you arch your

back, lifting your head and tailbone (Cow Pose). Exhale as you round your spine, tucking your chin and tailbone (Cat Pose). Move slowly and fluidly, synchronizing your breath with the movements.

2. Pelvic Tilts: Lie on your back with your knees bent and feet flat on the floor. Inhale to prepare, then exhale as you gently tilt your pelvis, pressing your lower back into the floor. Inhale to return to the starting position. This movement helps release tension in the lower back and hips.

3. Arm Circles: Stand or sit comfortably. Extend your arms out to the sides at shoulder height. Slowly make small circles with your arms, gradually increasing the size of the circles. Reverse the

direction after a minute. This exercise increases shoulder mobility and releases tension.

III. Awareness and Relaxation Practices:

Cultivating awareness and relaxation is a core component of somatic yoga, promoting a deeper connection between mind and body.

1. Body Scan Meditation: Lie down comfortably and close your eyes. Starting from your toes, mentally scan your body, noticing any areas of tension or discomfort. Breathe into these areas, allowing them to relax and release. Move slowly up through your body, finishing at the top of your head.

2. Progressive Muscle Relaxation: Sit or lie down comfortably. Starting with your feet, tense the muscles for a few seconds, then release and relax them. Move progressively up through your body, tensing and relaxing each muscle group. This technique helps release physical tension and promotes relaxation.

3. Mindful Movement: Perform simple movements, such as lifting your arms or stretching your legs, with full awareness. Pay attention to the sensations in your muscles and joints, the flow of your breath, and the feeling of the ground beneath you. Mindful movement enhances body awareness and mindfulness.

SOMATIC YOGA EXERCISES FOR BEGINNERS

Embarking on a somatic yoga journey can be a transformative experience, particularly when it comes to weight loss. Somatic yoga combines gentle movements with heightened body awareness, enabling you to re-educate your neuromuscular system and develop a deeper connection with your body. This chapter introduces four beginner-friendly somatic yoga exercises designed to enhance your practice and support your weight loss goals. Each exercise includes a detailed description, benefits, and step-by-step instructions.

Exercise 1: Pelvic Tilt:

I. Description and Benefits:

The pelvic tilt is a fundamental somatic yoga exercise that focuses on the lower back and pelvic region. It helps in relieving tension, improving flexibility, and strengthening the core muscles. This exercise is particularly beneficial for those who spend long hours sitting, as it promotes better posture and alleviates lower back pain. Additionally, the pelvic tilt enhances body awareness, allowing you to recognize and correct imbalances in your posture.

II. Step-by-Step Instructions:

1. Starting Position: Lie on your back with your knees bent and feet flat on the floor, hip-width apart.

Place your arms by your sides with your palms facing down.

2. Inhale: As you inhale, gently arch your lower back, creating a small space between your back and the floor. Feel the natural curve of your spine.

3. Exhale: As you exhale, slowly flatten your lower back against the floor by engaging your abdominal muscles. Tilt your pelvis upward, pressing your lower back into the mat.

4. Repeat: Perform this movement slowly and mindfully, inhaling to arch and exhaling to flatten. Repeat 10-15 times, focusing on the smooth, controlled movement of your pelvis.

Exercise 2: Cat-Cow Stretch:

I. Description and Benefits:

The Cat-Cow stretch is a dynamic somatic yoga exercise that improves spinal flexibility and relieves tension in the back, neck, and shoulders. This exercise helps in synchronizing breath with movement, promoting relaxation and reducing stress. Regular practice of the Cat-Cow stretch enhances body awareness and coordination, contributing to better posture and overall body alignment.

II. Step-by-Step Instructions:

1. Starting Position: Begin on your hands and knees in a tabletop position. Ensure your wrists are directly under your shoulders and your knees are under your hips.
2. **Inhale (Cow Pose):** As you inhale, drop your belly towards the

mat, lift your head and tailbone towards the ceiling, and arch your back. Allow your shoulder blades to move down your back.

3. Exhale (Cat Pose): As you exhale, tuck your chin to your chest, draw your belly button towards your spine, and round your back towards the ceiling. Press your hands and knees into the mat.

4. Repeat: Flow between Cat and Cow poses with each breath, inhaling to arch and exhaling to round. Continue for 1-2 minutes, moving slowly and mindfully.

Exercise 3: Shoulder Rolls:

I. Description and Benefits:

Shoulder rolls are a simple yet effective somatic yoga exercise that targets the shoulders and upper back. This exercise helps in releasing tension, improving shoulder mobility, and increasing blood circulation. Shoulder rolls also promote relaxation and body awareness, making them an excellent addition to any somatic yoga routine.

II. Step-by-Step Instructions:

1. Starting Position: Sit comfortably in a chair or on the floor with your back straight and shoulders relaxed. Place your hands on your thighs or knees.
2. Inhale: As you inhale, lift your shoulders up towards your ears, feeling the tension in your upper back and neck.
3. Exhale: As you exhale, roll your shoulders back and down,

squeezing your shoulder blades together. Feel the release of tension.

4. Repeat: Perform the shoulder rolls in a smooth, circular motion, inhaling to lift and exhaling to lower. Complete 10-15 rolls in one direction, then reverse the direction for another 10-15 rolls.

Exercise 4: Leg Slides:

I. Description and Benefits:

Leg slides are a gentle somatic yoga exercise that focuses on the lower body, particularly the hips, thighs, and lower back. This exercise helps in improving hip mobility, strengthening the core muscles, and enhancing body awareness. Leg slides are also beneficial for promoting relaxation and reducing tension in the lower body.

II. Step-by-Step Instructions:

1. Starting Position: Lie on your back with your legs extended and arms by your sides, palms facing down.

2. Inhale: As you inhale, slide your right heel along the floor towards your buttocks, bending your knee. Keep your foot in contact with the floor throughout the movement.

3. Exhale: As you exhale, slowly extend your right leg back to the starting position, sliding your heel along the floor.

4. Repeat: Perform the leg slide with your right leg 10-15 times, then switch to your left leg and repeat. Focus on the smooth,

controlled movement and the sensation in your lower body.

BUILDING YOUR SOMATIC YOGA ROUTINE

Creating an effective somatic yoga routine for weight loss involves more than just knowing the right exercises. It's about structuring your practice in a way that suits your lifestyle, meets your fitness goals, and can be adapted as you progress. This chapter will guide you through the essentials of building a personalized somatic yoga routine that maximizes your weight loss efforts and supports overall well-being.

A. Structuring Your Practice:

I. Frequency and Duration of Sessions:
To reap the full benefits of somatic yoga for weight loss, consistency is

key. Here are some guidelines to help you determine the optimal frequency and duration of your sessions:

1. Starting Out: If you're new to somatic yoga, aim for shorter sessions of about 20-30 minutes, 3-4 times a week. This allows your body to adapt gradually to the movements and techniques.

2. Building Consistency: As you become more comfortable, increase the duration of your sessions to 40-60 minutes. Strive to practice at least 4-5 times a week to maintain a steady rhythm and enhance your results.

3. Optimal Practice: For those who are committed to a significant weight loss journey, daily practice

of 60 minutes can be highly beneficial. Incorporate a mix of gentle and more intense sessions to keep your routine balanced and sustainable.

4. Rest and Recovery: While it's important to practice regularly, your body also needs time to recover. Ensure you include at least one rest day per week to prevent burnout and reduce the risk of injury.

II. Combining Exercises for a Balanced Routine:

A balanced somatic yoga routine should include a variety of exercises that address different aspects of fitness and well-being:

1. Warm-Up: Begin each session with gentle movements to increase blood flow and prepare your body for more intensive work. Simple stretches and breathing exercises can serve as an effective warm-up.

2. Core Practices: Include a mix of the following core somatic yoga exercises:
Cat-Cow Pose: Enhances spinal flexibility and strengthens the back and core.
Somatic Sun Salutations: A flowing sequence that combines stretching and strengthening.
Leg Lifts and Circles: Targets the lower body, aiding in muscle tone and flexibility.

3. Strength and Endurance: Incorporate poses that build strength and endurance, such as

Warrior Poses, Plank, and Bridge Pose. These exercises help in burning calories and building muscle mass, contributing to weight loss.

4. Cool-Down: End each session with a cool-down phase to help your body transition back to a resting state. Gentle stretches and relaxation techniques, such as Savasana (Corpse Pose), are ideal for cooling down.

5. Mindfulness and Breathing: Integrate mindfulness practices and breathwork throughout your session to enhance body awareness and promote stress reduction, both of which are crucial for weight loss.

 B. Adapting Exercises to Your Needs:

I. Modifications for Different Fitness Levels:

Somatic yoga is versatile and can be adapted to suit various fitness levels. Here's how you can modify exercises:

1. Beginners: Start with simplified versions of poses and use props such as yoga blocks, straps, or cushions to assist your movements. For example, if you find it challenging to maintain balance in Warrior Pose, use a chair for support.

2. Intermediate: As you gain strength and flexibility, gradually move to more advanced versions

of poses. Increase the duration you hold each pose and try variations that challenge your balance and coordination.

3. Advanced: For those with higher fitness levels, incorporate dynamic movements and hold poses for extended periods. Advanced practitioners can also explore more complex sequences that integrate multiple poses and transitions.

II. Progressing as You Improve:

Tracking your progress and adjusting your routine is crucial for continuous improvement and sustained weight loss:

1. Set Clear Goals: Define what you want to achieve with your

somatic yoga practice. Whether it's weight loss, improved flexibility, or better stress management, having clear goals will keep you motivated.

2. Monitor Your Progress: Keep a journal to track your sessions, noting any changes in your physical and mental well-being. Record the poses you practice, the duration, and any modifications you make.

3. Adjust Intensity: As your strength and endurance improve, gradually increase the intensity of your sessions. This could mean holding poses for longer, adding more repetitions, or incorporating new, more challenging poses.

4. Listen to Your Body: Pay attention to how your body responds to different exercises. If you experience discomfort or strain, adjust your practice accordingly. It's important to balance pushing your limits with respecting your body's signals.

5. Seek Guidance: Consider attending somatic yoga classes or consulting with a certified instructor, especially if you're unsure about how to progress safely. Professional guidance can help you refine your technique and ensure you're getting the most out of your practice.

ADVANCED SOMATIC YOGA TECHNIQUES

In this chapter, we delve into the advanced techniques of somatic yoga, aiming to deepen your practice and enhance its effectiveness for weight loss. We will explore more complex practices, advanced breathing techniques, and intricate movements and sequences. Additionally, we'll discuss how to seamlessly incorporate somatic yoga into your daily routine, even on the busiest of days, and how to integrate mindfulness and movement throughout your day.

A. Exploring Deeper Practices:

I. Advanced Breathing Techniques:

Breath is a cornerstone of somatic yoga, and mastering advanced breathing techniques can significantly enhance your practice and its benefits for weight loss.

1. Ujjayi Pranayama (Victorious Breath):
This breathing technique involves a slight constriction at the back of the throat, creating a soft, hissing sound. It promotes relaxation and enhances focus.

Practice:
Sit comfortably with a straight spine.
Inhale deeply through your nose, slightly constricting the back of your throat.
Exhale slowly, maintaining the constriction to create a soft sound.

Repeat for 5-10 minutes, focusing on the sound and sensation of your breath.

2. Kapalabhati (Skull Shining Breath):
This is an energizing breathing technique that involves forceful exhalations and passive inhalations. It stimulates the digestive system and can boost metabolism.

Practice:
Sit comfortably with a straight spine.
Take a deep breath in.
Exhale forcefully through your nose, drawing your navel toward your spine.
Allow the inhalation to be passive, then repeat the forceful exhalation.

Perform this for 1-2 minutes, gradually increasing the duration as you become more comfortable.

3. Nadi Shodhana (Alternate Nostril Breathing):
This balancing breathing technique calms the mind and balances the body's energy channels, aiding in stress reduction and promoting overall well-being.

Practice:
Sit comfortably with a straight spine.
Use your right thumb to close your right nostril.
Inhale deeply through your left nostril.
Close your left nostril with your right ring finger, then release your right nostril and exhale through it.

Inhale through your right nostril, then close it with your thumb.
Release your left nostril and exhale through it.
Continue this pattern for 5-10 minutes.

II. More Complex Movements and Sequences:

As you progress in your somatic yoga practice, integrating more complex movements and sequences can challenge your body and mind, enhancing your physical fitness and body awareness.

1. Somatic Sun Salutations:
A variation of the traditional sun salutation sequence, incorporating mindful, slow movements, and breath awareness.

Practice:

Begin in Tadasana (Mountain Pose).

Inhale, reach your arms overhead, and gently arch back.

Exhale, fold forward into Uttanasana (Forward Bend).

Inhale, lift halfway, elongating your spine.

Exhale, step back into a plank position.

Lower into Chaturanga Dandasana (Low Plank) with control.

Inhale, transition into Bhujangasana (Cobra Pose).

Exhale, move into Adho Mukha Svanasana (Downward-Facing Dog).

Inhale, step forward into Uttanasana.

Exhale, rise back up to Tadasana.

Repeat this sequence 3-5 times, focusing on smooth, mindful movements.

2. Dynamic Somatic Sequences:
These sequences combine multiple poses in fluid, continuous movements, enhancing strength, flexibility, and coordination.

Practice:
Start in Warrior II (Virabhadrasana II).
Transition into Reverse Warrior, then into Extended Side Angle Pose (Utthita Parsvakonasana).
Flow into Triangle Pose (Trikonasana), then into Half Moon Pose (Ardha Chandrasana).
Return to Warrior II, and repeat on the opposite side.

Perform this sequence slowly, paying attention to alignment and breath.

B. Incorporating Somatic Yoga into Daily Life:

I. Short Practices for Busy Days:

Even on the busiest days, short somatic yoga practices can provide significant benefits, helping you stay grounded and focused.

1. Morning Routine:
A quick 10-minute practice to energize your body and mind for the day ahead.

Practice:
Begin with 2-3 minutes of Ujjayi Pranayama.

Move through a brief sequence of cat-cow stretches, seated twists, and gentle forward bends.
End with a short meditation, focusing on your breath and setting a positive intention for the day.

2. Lunchtime Reset:
A mid-day practice to refresh and re-energize.

Practice:
Start with 2-3 minutes of Kapalabhati breathing.
Perform a few standing poses like Warrior I and II, and gentle backbends like Camel Pose.
Finish with a short body scan meditation, releasing any tension.

3. Evening Unwind:

A calming practice to help you relax and prepare for sleep.

Practice:
Begin with 2-3 minutes of Nadi Shodhana.
Move through gentle seated stretches like Janu Sirsasana (Head-to-Knee Pose) and Supine Twist.
Conclude with a 5-minute Savasana, focusing on deep, relaxed breathing.

II. Integrating Mindfulness and Movement Throughout the Day:

Incorporating mindfulness and movement into your daily routine can enhance your somatic yoga practice and overall well-being.

1. Mindful Walking:

Turn your daily walks into a mindful practice by focusing on each step, the sensations in your body, and your breath.

Practice:
As you walk, pay attention to the contact of your feet with the ground.
Notice the movement of your legs and the swing of your arms.
Sync your breath with your steps, creating a rhythmic flow.

2. Desk Yoga:
Integrate somatic movements and stretches into your workday to alleviate tension and improve posture.

Practice:

Take a few minutes every hour to stretch your arms, shoulders, and neck.
Perform seated twists and forward bends to release tension in your back.
Practice deep, mindful breathing to reduce stress and increase focus.

3. Bedtime Routine:
End your day with a few gentle stretches and mindful breathing to promote relaxation and improve sleep quality.

Practice:
Lie on your back and gently hug your knees to your chest.
Perform gentle supine twists to release any remaining tension.

Finish with a few minutes of deep, relaxed breathing, focusing on letting go of the day's stresses.

By incorporating these advanced techniques and integrating somatic yoga into your daily life, you can deepen your practice, enhance your body awareness, and support your weight loss journey in a holistic and sustainable way.

COMBINING SOMATIC YOGA WITH OTHER WEIGHT LOSS STRATEGIES

In our journey toward achieving weight loss and overall well-being, it's essential to understand that no single strategy stands alone. While somatic yoga offers incredible benefits for weight loss through neuromuscular re-education, stress reduction, and enhanced body awareness, combining it with other weight loss strategies can amplify these effects. This chapter delves into the synergy between somatic yoga and other key components such as nutrition, mindful eating, and complementary physical activities.

A. Nutrition and Somatic Awareness:

I. Mindful Eating Practices:

Mindful eating is a practice that encourages us to be present during meals, paying full attention to the experience of eating. This involves recognizing physical hunger and fullness cues, savoring each bite, and eating without distractions. When combined with somatic yoga, mindful eating can transform the way we approach food, helping us make healthier choices and develop a better relationship with eating.

1. Recognizing Hunger and Fullness Cues: Somatic yoga enhances our body awareness, making it easier to distinguish between true hunger and emotional cravings. Practicing mindful eating involves taking a

moment to assess our hunger levels before reaching for food and stopping when we feel comfortably full.

2. Savoring Each Bite: Engage your senses by noticing the colors, textures, and flavors of your food. Chew slowly and thoroughly, allowing yourself to fully experience each bite. This not only improves digestion but also prevents overeating.

3. Eating Without Distractions: In our fast-paced world, it's common to eat while working, watching TV, or scrolling through our phones. Mindful eating encourages us to create a calm environment for meals, free from distractions. This practice helps us stay present and fully enjoy our food.

II. Healthy Eating Tips:

Incorporating healthy eating habits is crucial for weight loss and overall health. Here are some tips that align well with the principles of somatic yoga:

1. Balanced Diet: Aim for a diet rich in whole foods, including fruits, vegetables, lean proteins, whole grains, and healthy fats. Avoid processed foods and sugary snacks, which can lead to weight gain and negatively impact your energy levels.

2. Portion Control: Be mindful of portion sizes to avoid overeating. Using smaller plates and bowls can help you manage portions better. Pay attention to your

body's signals and stop eating when you feel satisfied.

3. Stay Hydrated: Drinking plenty of water throughout the day is essential for maintaining proper hydration and supporting metabolic processes. Sometimes, our bodies can mistake thirst for hunger, leading to unnecessary snacking.

4. Regular Meal Times: Establish regular eating patterns by having meals and snacks at consistent times each day. This helps regulate your metabolism and prevents the urge to overeat.

B. Complementary Physical Activities:
In addition to somatic yoga, engaging in complementary

physical activities can further support your weight loss journey. These activities provide variety, enhance fitness levels, and prevent exercise monotony.

I. Walking, Swimming, and Other Low-Impact Exercises:

Low-impact exercises are gentle on the joints while effectively burning calories and improving cardiovascular health. They can be easily integrated with somatic yoga to create a balanced fitness routine.

1. Walking: Walking is a simple yet powerful exercise that can be done anywhere. It helps improve cardiovascular health, burn calories, and reduce stress. Incorporating mindful walking,

where you pay attention to your breath and surroundings, can further enhance the benefits.

2. Swimming: Swimming is an excellent full-body workout that is easy on the joints. It improves cardiovascular fitness, builds muscle strength, and enhances flexibility. The soothing nature of water can also have a calming effect, complementing the relaxation achieved through somatic yoga.

3. Cycling: Whether on a stationary bike or outdoors, cycling is a low-impact exercise that improves cardiovascular health and leg strength. It's an enjoyable way to stay active and can be adjusted to various intensity levels.

II. Strength Training and Flexibility Exercises:

Building muscle and improving flexibility are essential components of a balanced fitness routine. These exercises complement somatic yoga by enhancing overall body strength, stability, and mobility.

1. Strength Training: Incorporating strength training exercises, such as weight lifting or bodyweight exercises (e.g., push-ups, squats, lunges), helps build lean muscle mass. Increased muscle mass boosts metabolism, aiding in weight loss. Strength training also improves bone density and joint health.

2. Flexibility Exercises: Stretching and flexibility exercises, such as those found in Pilates or dedicated stretching routines, improve range of motion and reduce the risk of injury. These exercises can be seamlessly integrated with somatic yoga to enhance body awareness and relaxation.

CONCLUSION

Reflecting on Your Journey:

As you reach the end of this book, it's important to take a moment to reflect on the journey you've embarked upon. Somatic yoga is not just a practice but a lifestyle that fosters a deep connection between your mind and body. By now, you've likely experienced the transformative power of somatic yoga, witnessing changes not only in your weight but also in your overall well-being.

Tracking Progress and Celebrating Milestones:

One of the key aspects of any journey, especially one as personal as weight loss and self-improvement, is tracking your progress. Keeping a journal or a log of your experiences, challenges, and victories can provide a tangible record of how far you've come. Celebrate every milestone, no matter how small. Whether it's reaching a certain weight, mastering a challenging pose, or simply feeling more at peace with your body, each step forward is a testament to your dedication and hard work. These celebrations fuel your motivation and remind you that progress is a series of small, consistent steps.

Staying Motivated and Committed to Your Practice:

Staying motivated can sometimes be challenging, especially when faced with obstacles or slow progress. Remember why you started this journey. Revisit the goals you set and the reasons behind them. Surround yourself with supportive individuals, whether it's a community of fellow practitioners, friends, or family. Engage with content that inspires you, be it books, videos, or stories of others who have walked a similar path. Consistency is key, and even on days when motivation wanes, the discipline of showing up and practicing can sustain your progress and commitment.

Future Directions:

Your journey with somatic yoga doesn't end here. In fact, this is just the beginning. The principles and practices you've learned can continue to evolve and grow with you, adapting to your changing needs and goals.

Continuing to Grow and Evolve with Somatic Yoga:

As you move forward, consider exploring advanced techniques and poses that challenge and expand your practice. Attend workshops or retreats to deepen your understanding and connect with other practitioners. Keep abreast of new research and developments in the field of somatic yoga and weight loss, integrating new findings into your routine. Personal growth is a continuous journey, and somatic yoga offers a rich, lifelong path to health, mindfulness, and self-discovery.

In conclusion, somatic yoga is a powerful tool for weight loss and overall wellness. By reflecting on your journey, celebrating your achievements, and staying motivated, you can sustain the benefits you've gained. Embrace the future with an open mind, and let somatic yoga continue to guide you towards a healthier, more balanced life. Thank you for allowing this book to be a part of your journey. May your practice be ever enriching and your progress ever rewarding.

THE END